12 Quick Marketing Ideas for Dentists:

No-cost or low-cost real-life tips, except one of them

DR. GERMAN GOMEZ

D.D.S., M.D., Ph.D.

DEDICATION

To my beautiful daughter and wife, who support me every day. Their unconditional love is my biggest strength.

To my parents and brothers, whose constant faith, hope, help, and love have been a pillar for me through the peaks and valleys of my life's journey

TABLE OF CONTENT

ACKNOWLEDGMENTS

The contents of this work are intended to further general understanding and discussion only, and are not intended and should not be relied upon as recommending or promoting a specific method, diagnosis, or treatment by health science practitioners for any particular patient. The author makes no representations or warranties with respect to the accuracy or completeness of the contents of this work and specifically disclaims all warranties, including without limitation any implied warranties for a particular purpose. Given ongoing research, equipment modifications, changes in governmental regulations, and the constant flow of information relating to the use of medicines, equipment, and devices, the reader is urged to review and evaluate the information provided. Readers should consult with a specialist where appropriate. The fact that an organization or Website is referred to in this work as a citation and/or a potential source of further information does not mean that the author or the publisher endorses the information the organization or Website may provide or recommendations it may make. Further, readers should be aware that Internet Websites listed in this work may have changed or disappeared between when this work was written and when it is read. No warranty may be created or extended by any promotional statements for this work. The author shall not be liable for any damages arising therefrom.

Last but not least, when the author is writing about, and referring himself to the patient, the dentist or the dental team as "he", or is using the male version in an example, his intention is always to include the male, female and diverse genders.

1
INTRODUCTION

Dear reader, thank you for buying this book. It is directed to dentists the staff of the office, and everybody who wants to improve the service to their patients.

If your clinical skills are excellent, but you want more patients to come to your office and start recommending you and your staff, then this book is the right one for you.

You will be equipped with real-world tips on It gives you real-life tips on some ideas for marketing for dentists and dental offices.

You will learn, among other things what your Sales Funnel is, how to put together packages and menus, a Fishbowl-Idea, how to award patients, a wedding strategy, and special Marketing procedures.

It is NOT meant to be a comprehensive marketing guide for dentists, but just a small collection of ideas you can implement easily and very quickly in your office. These ideas have given our office real boosts in terms of new patient acquisition and sales.

Some chapters of this book are also part of other books that I have written. I repeat them here, as it makes sense for the overall understanding of the concepts and processes. So that this book can also stand alone as a comprehensive work by itself.

This book is tailored for dentists. But it also applies to office managers, office administrators, front desk employees, and their teams.

The moment you opened up a dental office, you started to be in business. You have all these expenses that you have to cover every month, your staff, your loans, your rent, everything.

Without a business attitude, you will not be successful. Although you might only compete against other dentists in your field and although you might not be in a country where real businessmen and businesswomen are involved in the dental business.

Also, if you are only competing against other dentists, it's not a bad idea to have all the setup and processes in place to give your patients an extraordinary experience they will remember.

These processes are given to you with books like this. Or you have an ability by yourself and you develop these ideas through time.

So, this is what we did. I am condensing these tips, that have helped us, for you in this book.

I hope you enjoy this book and you get a lot of ideas, interesting ideas, and you improve your results.

Thank you again for reading this book, I hope you enjoy it and that it provides you with some advanced knowledge and ideas.

2
YOUR SALES FUNNEL

In this chapter, we will talk about your sales funnel.

It is the process of getting people into your office and then offering them a really good treatment.

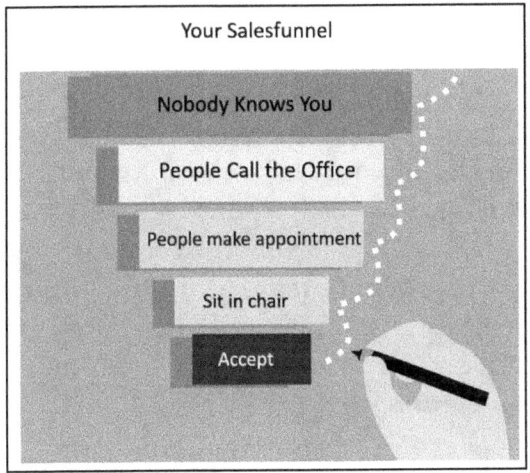

Steps:
1. Make them aware
2. Make them schedule an appointment
3. Make them sit in the chair
4. Make them accept the treatment plan

Step 1: Make them aware

In the beginning, nobody knows you. As nobody knew me in Valencia in Spain, nobody.

So you have to make people aware that you exist. How do you do that? With marketing, ads, and so on.

So, here is the activity of marketing in between the block "Nobody knows you" and the block "People contact the office". They can call, they can write an email, they can go to your website and subscribe to your newsletter, they can come to your office, walk in and ask for information.

Step 2: Make them schedule an appointment

People are now aware, then, once they call, you have to be aware, that not everybody who calls makes an appointment. Who is there to make that person, that calls, schedule an appointment?

Your front office. Your front office has to be trained in sales skills and in communication skills to make the most of this situation. If the front office is skillful, most of these people make an appointment in your office.

Step 3: Make them sit in the chair

Then from an appointment, some of them will pull back. They will just not come. Who is responsible for that? Still, the front office. That is why the front office training and front office management are very important.

Avoiding these no-shows is crucial and does not depend at all on the clinical skills of the dentist or the team. It is just a skill more in the repertoire of the front desk.

Step 3: Make them accept the treatment plan

Once they sit in the chair and you present, for example, a very comprehensive implants treatment in combination with veneers and crowns, and bridges. Now the patient has to accept that.

Here it's you as a dentist, your communication skill, and your sales skill. But also the team's skills, as all comments, and reinforcements count. Your front office can still make or break the acceptance when she gives the next schedule or when he or she explains the financial issues.

It is important that you know exactly the numbers. You have to know the number of new patients calling or contacting the office in different ways. Such as by email, website chats, WhatsApp, through your Social Media or just walking into the office and asking a question. Patients who contact your office because of word of mouth or because of your advertisement, your marketing, and your online or offline marketing.

People that contact your office for information, then, apart from this number, you need to know how many of these people you have actually seen in your office.

That means how many of these new patient contacts are converted into new patients seen in your office.

Then, from these new patients that you see, how many of these new patients really make the treatment with you?

These are patients that say yes to your treatment options, who have paid, and the work is done. What is the number?

In the sales funnel, you measure how many you convert in every step. You need to know all these figures. If you have these data you know what and where you can improve something.

It's extremely important to have very good communication skills to run a successful dental office.

3
DIFFERENCE BETWEEN MARKETING VS SALES & FEATURES VS BENEFITS

What is marketing?

Well, in one sentence, marketing is everything you do, to bring a patient into your office, to make him call you, to make him contact you.

Marketing is everything you do to bring a patient in.
Advertisement,
offers,
your office design is also marketing,
the way you dress,
social media,
your website,
your logo,
business card stationery, that means your letterhead, a.s.o.
Your location is marketing,
front office protocols,
how they pick up the phone in your office,
how they answer the phone,
how they get the calls, and so on.
All the protocols in the front office.
Positioning of your advertisements,
also positioning of your clinic location,
your branding is marketing your message.
How you communicate your message out there.

Social proof is marketing.

Real reputation is marketing and so many things.

Sales is different.

Sales is everything you do face to face. If the patient is already in.

How is your office structured?

What's the first contact when the patient is in your office?

How is your front desk treating him?

How is your reception area?

How is the protocol for the first patient visit?

All these things are already sales.

How you inform the patient about the treatment options.

How you convince the patient to choose one or another treatment.

How you close the treatment, your closing techniques.

How you present the case to them.

Your communication skills, that show your empathy.

How you listen to what the patient says and how you later take it into your case presentation or your communication. All this is sales.

When your marketing is good, the less sales you have to do. You have already sold by your good marketing, by the way, you get them in. For example, if you use social media, this is selling for you while it gets you patients in. If the marketing is very, very good, it's easy for you to open that shell later on during the sales process.

Feature versus benefit.

A feature is, what something does or has. For example, a crown rebuilds and covers a tooth.

Bleaching whitens teeth. That is a feature of bleaching.

Periodontal treatment: the feature is, that it cleans up the pockets.

A crown is made out of ceramic Emax™, zircon, name it, that's a feature. Another feature would be, that it is a very hard crown.

Bleaching with a lamp or without a lamp.

Bleaching with 32% of hydrogen peroxide.

Periodontal treatment with laser, open or closed scaling, and root planing.

The benefit is what it does for the patient. What does it do for him? What is the treatment of a crown doing for him? He can now chew without fear to break a tooth or something like that. Or he can smile without fear.

Bleaching: smiling the bright way. That's a benefit for the patient.

Periodontal treatment: no gum bleeding anymore, or no bad breath anymore. That's a benefit of periodontal treatment.

What you want to do is in your marketing and sales message: you want to concentrate on the benefits, not on the features.

What's in it for him?

What does it do for the patient?

- Create awareness of your patient's problem and then show how the benefit of your treatment can help.

IDEAS

4
IDEA #1: DON´T BE CHEAP

It's the value, it's not the price.

If you look at your competitors and only look at the price, what is usually charged for certain procedures in the market, for example, what does a crown/whitening/implant cost?

I ask you: If you do that, who is determining your price then? Answer: The other dentists! So, you take the mean value of the other dentists. Does this decide upon your price? That's not possible, that should not be true.

First of all, your price should cover all your expenses and give you a profit. Of course, your expenses are not the same as in other clinics, so it should not be a habit to look at the market prices to establish your own price. This does not make sense at so many levels. Calculate your overhead costs per hour and then add the specific hourly costs per procedure and add a profit margin.

YOU have to decide your price. And you have to create your price. Not lower, higher.

If somebody had come to me 25/30 years ago and had said to me: "I have a very good idea. But I need some money from you. Please lend me 5000 euros". I had asked: "For what kind of business?". That person would have answered: "I have the best business idea ever". And then this guy tells me about his idea. His idea is to make a coffee shop. But instead of asking 50 cents for the coffee, he will ask $3 for the coffee. That's his idea. And then I would say: "What?? I will not give you the 5000 euros, you're silly". So in this hypothetical example, the founder of Starbucks™ was asking me for $5,000 to get into his business. And I would have definitely said no, 25/30 years ago.

Now we know, this would have been the business of my life. So, it's not the price, people look at the value and the value is personal. It has nothing to do with the price.

You have to put up your value. The value is composed out of your brand, your communication skills, your sales skills, how you act in front of the patient, and your environment, the technology you use. You can also explain to the patient, that you use the best dental technicians and the best materials. And he has to see and understand all that also. It is not only about telling him but also about proof.

All that makes you more valuable than other dentists. So your price can be higher than other dentists.

Work on your brand, work on all the skills I just mentioned, and work on the environment. This will give you and your work a much higher value, and then you can charge more for your service.

The fact, that you charge more is in itself a marketing measure, as it also automatically gives your brand a higher value. That is the basic idea not to be cheap as a marketing idea.

5
IDEA #2: PUT "PACKAGES" TOGETHER

What is a package? Well, it's something that can make a treatment much more valuable. Patients obviously want value for their money.

Try to set your procedure fee as a package deal and show them the true value of your offer. Imagine a Fläsh procedure.

Setting your Fees
- Patients want value for their money
- Try setting your fee as a **"Package Deal"** and show the **true value** of what you offer

Our Fläsh Procedure Fee includes:
- – Free plaque removal on the day of Bleaching — 40$
- – Whitening Procedure — 760$
- – Custom-fitted trays — 250 $
- – Post care Take-Home Whitening Gel — 150 $

Whitening Package: $525!
Valued at $1,200

Free plaque removal on the day of bleaching. You take away, not the tartar, but the pellicle, you know, just a little bit, you brush the teeth with a polish paste before the whitening.

You could say: "I do that anyhow". I know you do that, but put a price on it. Imagine somebody comes to your office and says: "Doctor, I want you to brush my teeth with a polishing paste, but I will do the whitening with somebody else". In this case, what would you charge for that brushing of the teeth? Put the price on it.

Then the whitening procedure itself. Put a price on it a little bit higher than you would usually charge for it.

Then custom-fitted trays that you do for the patient. Although he makes an in-office whitening, he gets trays. These are not meant to be for home bleaching, they may be used for desensitizing in very sensible patients. He may use these trays for a touch-up a year from now, or so.

And then he also gets a take-home whitening syringe. Post-care take-home whitening gel.

You might say: "But I do the trays anyhow". I know you do the trays. But imagine again, a patient comes to your office and says I want you to make me some trays, but I will do the actual whitening with another dentist. What would you charge for the trays? Put the price on it. And imagine the patient comes in and says "I want one of these touch-up gels, but I will do the bleaching with another dentist", what would you charge? Put that on the price list.

So you calculate the price list and all that together has a value of $1,200. But you give all this together away for $525.

Now you will say: "But all the dentists do all these services inside of a whitening procedure". Yes, but not all dentists explain to the patient that it's not only a whitening. It is much more than a whitening. And it has a much, much higher value than what you actually asked for a simple whitening.

That is the trick. So put together some packages.

6
IDEA #3: OFFER MENU-OPTIONS

Idea number three, offer menu options.

What is a menu option? For example, Starbucks™ has all the combinations that they can do in coffees, with ice, without ice with a little bit of milk, with soy milk, with almond milk, and with all kinds of different options. If you calculate all these options, they have 10,000 different products they can offer to you as one coffee.

Now you cannot make people be confused about your offers. You can narrow it down to three offers for example. Let me explain it to you here for example in a whitening:

Type		Product	Method	Procedure includes	Price
In- Office		with lamp	one session in the office about 1 hour	-Plaque removal -Fläsh procedure 32% -Trays -Post-treatment	X €
Combined		combined lamp and take-home	1 hour in-office + 1 week at home	-Plaque removal -Fläsh procedure 6% -Trays -Post-treatment -Take-home gel	X €
Take-Home		individual tray	2 weeks at home	-Plaque removal -Trays -Take-home gel	X €

15

You can have an in-office whitening, you can have a combined whitening, in-office and take-home, and you can have a take-home whitening offer for the patient.

And all these three options have different prices. Now you have to explain to the patient, through the menu, not yourself, what the difference is.

Well, one is done with a lamp, the other is a lamp and take home, and the third one is done with individual trays, only, to take home.

The first option is one session in the office in about one hour. The second option is one hour in the office and one week at home and the third option is two weeks at home.

The combined has a less strong in-office gel. The in-office treatment has a 32% Hydrogen Peroxide, but the combined option has only 6% Hydrogen Peroxide. That's why you have to whiten at home still all the nights during one week. So, one hour in the office and then one week at home instead of two weeks if you don't make the in-office step. These are the three options in our example.

So, people who don't like in-office whitening because they have very sensitive teeth, have now two other options. There is a faster option or a slower option.

I give you another example. You can do the same thing with implants. Just work with three different brands, for example. Or with three different options of the same brand.

choose YOUR IMPLANT	STANDARD € implant + met.-cer. crown	PROFESSIONAL € implant + met.-cer. crown	LUXURY € implant + met.-cer. crown
KEY FEATURES			
Origin of the Implant	Corea	European Union	European Union
ISO and CE - Certificates	✓	✓	✓
Guarante - all components	4 years	7 years	7 years
Scientific background	-	✓	✓
CAD-CAM components	-	✓	✓
× 30 years research	-	-	✓
CROWNS			
Dental Lab	European Union	European Union	European Union
High Esthetic Crown	-	✓	✓
UPGRADES			
Zirconium-Ceramic Crown	+ 150 €	+ 150 €	+ 150 €

So you can put a menu together. In this example, the different options are called, standard option, professional option, and luxury option. You can name them however you like.

And they have different prices, the luxury option is nearly three times more than the standard option. And the professional option is nearly double. It's like, Economy Class, Business class, and First class. Usually, people understand these examples.

Why do you have an economy, a business, and a first class? If you fly from Frankfurt to Dubai, all three classes get to Dubai. So all three here are implants. But there are differences.

What is the difference? Maybe the origin of the implant. In one case, it is Korea, and in the other two cases, it is the European Union. All of them have ISO and CE certificates.

You can also give different guarantees. That's up to you, you give the guarantee. So you say, I give only four years of guarantee for the economy or the standard option, then I give seven years of guarantee for the professional or business class implant, and you can go up to 10 years for the luxury.

Then you can say, that two of them have a scientific background, two of them have CAD/CAM components, but only one of them has more than 30 years of research.

And then the crowns. You just don't make a very high aesthetic crown on the economy class, which means you use a dental technician, who is a low-price and low-aesthetic technician.

You can also have upgrades on all of them.

You see the differences, just put a menu together so that people are aware of what options they have in your office. That is internal marketing, by the way. And you can publish it on social media, you can publish it on your website, and then it's not only internal marketing, it is converted into external marketing, too. Not a lot of dentists have that. This makes you appear different.

7
IDEA #4: THE "FISHBOWL" COLLECTION

Now, idea number four. I call it the fishbowl collection.

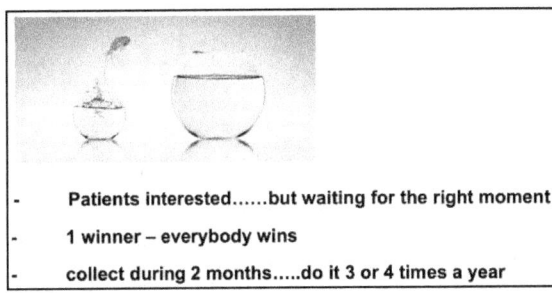

- Patients interested......but waiting for the right moment
- 1 winner – everybody wins
- collect during 2 months.....do it 3 or 4 times a year

I have this fishbowl in my office in the reception area. There is no water in it, and there is no fish in it. And right next to this fishbowl, there is a sign.

And this sign says: "Do you want to win a free whitening? Fill out this paper".

There is a sheet of paper where the patient can put in their name, his or her email address, and mobile number. This paper also has a data release form, that they have to sign. And then they put that paper in the bowl and I leave it there for two months for example. After two months, I just take one paper out and this is the winner and he or she gets a free whitening.

Usually, they get a take-home whitening, but if the patient wants to upgrade to an in-office whitening, he can do that. He just pays the difference.

There is one winner, but in the end, everybody wins. So I will contact all of these patients because I know these patients want a whitening. But why haven't they made a whitening already? They have not made a whitening already, because they are waiting for the right moment to do it.

The right moment for them is, when it is cheap. The best moment is, when it is for free, of course. And the second best moment is, when there is a very good offer.

So I contact all of these patients, and I say to them: "Such a pity you did not win the free whitening. But I have good news for you, if you call today, (or if you call in the next 48 hours or 24 hours or whatever), then you can have a whitening with a 30% discount (20% discount, 50% discount, whatever you think it's okay for you).

You most probably will convert a lot of these patients, who are interested in whitening (otherwise they would not have taken part in the raffle) to real whitening patients.

You can also ask the patients to fill out the paper for friends and family, with the respective data (there you have to be careful, as data protection laws may apply in your country), and maybe they win a free whitening.

So they fill out the name, the phone number in the email address of their friends and families. Like this, I get new leads, I get new people to contact. And I will contact them, telling them that one of my patients (and I tell them the name) wanted something good for them and wanted them to win a free whitening, but they did not win it.

Well, if they won it, then, of course, they won it, but only one person wins. So most of them will not. I will contact them anyhow and tell them about the offer. And then maybe they come into the office, most of them do that.

8
IDEA #5: YOU SHOULD AWARD PATIENTS

Award the patient if he brings you new patients in. That is also marketing.

You can give the patient a whitening touch-up for free if he brings in one or two new patients to whiten their teeth.

This referring patient, for example, makes his bleaching and after one year he comes to his control and his prophylaxis, and he says "My teeth are a little bit yellowish. I would like to have a touch-up, a refreshment". What you can say is: "I can give that to you for free. If you bring one (or two or three, whatever) new patient(s), who will make a whitening procedure in this office, then you get that for free".

This is an offer that you make for the patient. Another possibility is, that if he brings 10 patients in, he gets a whole whitening for free, which he can gift to another patient if he had already done a whitening on his teeth just a short time ago.

Another idea is to award your patient with a discount voucher of 10, 20, 30…. Euros, depending on how much the new patient he brought in, spent in treatments in your office.

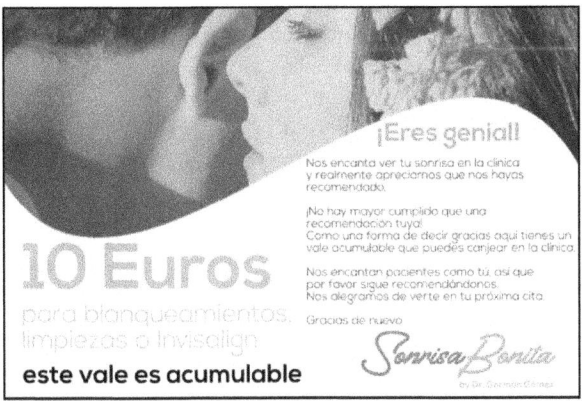

These vouchers can be spent for bleaching for a cleaning, prophylaxis and for Invisalign.

Above these lines, you see an example of a 10 Euros voucher. It says:

"10 Euros for whitening, cleanings, or Invisalign.

You are great!

We love to see your smile at our office and we really appreciate that you have recommended us.

There is no higher compliment than your recommendation!

As a way of saying thank you here is a cumulative voucher that you can exchange at the office.

We love patients like you, so please keep recommending us.

We are glad to see you at your next appointment.

Thanks again"

So, he can spend that in our office. And the more patients he refers, the more vouchers he has, and the more vouchers he can redeem, but only in whitening, cleanings, and invisible aligners. Usually the margins are big enough in these treatments, that you can make these things. You can make a 10 Euro discount without any problems in these treatments.

9
IDEA #6: DO VIDEO MARKETING

In this chapter, I will write about why and how dentists should do video marketing.

You will learn why it is better than other methods and marketing strategies, how to structure an up to 10 minutes video, when to upload it, how to structure a YouTube video ad, and how to find a good title for your video.

Video marketing is attraction marketing. But there are other types of marketing like interruption marketing, in the malls.

Interruption marketing: When you go to a mall and there is a booth with credit cards or so and they stop you. You're going to go somewhere else but they stop you and they ask you: do you have a credit card? And that is annoying.

Also on Facebook™, you find interruption marketing: sponsored ads. You are reading the posts of your friends and families, and of the groups, you are in, and all of a sudden there are some sponsored ads. That's annoying.

Attraction marketing is when someone is looking up something, and your video comes up on YouTube™ or Google™, or somewhere else.

Here's a template for a 10 minutes video.

- Start. The first five seconds are all about grabbing attention maybe with a question. You have to say: Hey, I'm here. That's grabbing attention.

- The next 10 to 15 seconds are to introduce yourself and reveal the main benefits of the video. Why should they watch this video?

- and then you should make an opener logo for 10 to 15 seconds. For example, you can go to the websites of videohive.net for some introduction videos, you just put your logo into that, and audiojungle.net is for music that you can buy and then put it as background for this logo-introduction-video.

- After that, the main content, it's two to seven minutes. It depends on what content you want to show. You want to show how to brush your teeth, you brush your teeth. You want to show how to floss, you show that. Do you want to show how to scrape your tongue or how the experience is, the first time a patient comes to the office? You make a video about that.

- Then, in the end, you have to have a call to action. Maybe one, that people should subscribe to your channel, watch more videos, ask questions or they should call a number and come to your office or visit your website. What do you want people to do after they watch the video?

- Then the final exit video. Listing your social media or

something like that. You can also go to videohive and look for templates of that to upload.

Statistics have shown, that the best time to upload a video is Tuesdays at 9 am.

The second choice would be Thursdays at the same time.

The third best option is Wednesdays or Fridays also the same time.

Here's a template for a video for a YouTube™ ad.

- In the first five seconds, you grab attention maybe with a question,

- then you talk about the pain points, and their struggle, and talk about feelings on how you will make them feel. How good they feel before the treatment and after the treatment.

- And the solution. You try to give them a view of the solution. You show them, that you have the solution for the bad feelings they are in now (either real or provoked by putting a seed in their mind with your question at the beginning) and how they get to the good feeling after the treatment. This treatment helps you to do this and that or to have this and that. For example, this periodontal treatment helps you to get rid of your bleeding in the gums and to have fresh breath. Or to get rid of your pain, if the pain point is bad breath.

- Then a call to action. What do you want people to do after they watch the video?

- And then the final exit video, social media like 10 seconds to show, that you are on social media, that you have a Facebook site, that you have a web page, and so on.

Tips on how to find a good title for your video. As for advertisements, you have to have the same strategy.

- Stated as a question. Do you want to...? or Would you like to...? Do you want to learn how to brush your teeth thoroughly? or Do you want to know how the first-time experience in our office is? Would you like to see a patient's experience the first time he comes into our office?

- State it as a secret. For example: Secrets on how to get rid of snoring at night. Then you can talk about all your sleep dentistry devices or treatments.

Make it newsy. Introducing, announcing, discovering. For example, "Announcing the new ceramic dental implant". Then you talk about new implants you've bought and how you will put them into the patients.

10
IDEA #7: STRATEGIC GIVE-AWAYS

What does that mean? Imagine your dealer in your country makes a good offer, maybe a 20% discount on whitening kits. Well, then you take advantage of this deal, imagine a "buy five get one free"-deal.

But you don't go down 20% with your price. So you buy 10 and get two kits for free. You give these free whitenings away to strategically chosen people, not to your best friend.

Who are the strategic key persons for your office? Makeup specialists, stylists, hairstylists, trainers in gyms, celebrities in your town, celebrity representatives, influencers in your town, stewardesses, hostesses, and receptionists in hotels.

Let me give you an example. You want to be known as one of the top dentists in town. So, you go to the most expensive, makeup specialist and stylist in town. And you enter there and you say "Hello, I'm Dr. X, who is the boss here?". They will tell you who the responsible person there is. Then I go up to him or her. Usually, the boss is the owner and is not a worker there. You want to talk to the owner.

You say to the owner: " Hello, I'm Dr. X, I have a good offer for you so that we can cooperate". The first reaction these owners usually have is to decline your offer, although they still have not even heard the offer. "I'm not interested". That's what they all say. "Not interested, go home. I don't care about what you want to say to me".

Then you say " I will give you a bleaching for free for yourself. If you sit down with me and we will have a chat. I will bleach your teeth and we make your teeth white for free". This offer usually opens the door. "Oh, do you want a coffee? Do you want to sit down? Come in". All of a sudden, it's okay.

So, you sit down with the owner. And then you say to the owner: "I want to make also a whitening for free for your best employee here". The best employee in a makeup studio, fingernails specialists, and all these things. This best employee usually is chatting the whole time with the clients. Who are these clients? Because it's the most expensive studio in town, are usually the richest women in town. These women go to these specialists. And these richest women are chatting the whole time with the girl that makes the fingernails and make-up eyebrows, you know.

You say to the boss: "I want to make a free whitening also for her and we will tell her that you pay for this whitening". Immediately the owner, who could be confused, says: "I will not pay anything". You answer: "No, no, you will not pay anything. I will pay for it. But we will tell her that you paid for it". The owner then usually asks: "Why would you do that?". You answer: "Because I want her to think you are a good boss".

In the end, I will make a free whitening on the best employee, the one who talks a lot to the clients and everybody wants to be with her. All the rich ladies want to go to her. She's the best one. She is the one. And she comes into our office. And the moment that she comes into your office. She's not aware of it, but I am training her in selling whitening. I am explaining to her everything. My team is explaining her everything she needs to know about whitening, and how to explain whitening to others. To whom? To the rich ladies.

And then we make her also aware that she now looks really nice and beautiful. And next time she is working. She has another attitude. She is smiling even more. And while she is talking, the rich ladies notice something different. "What happened? You look different today." And then she says: "Well, I made a whitening with Dr. X". Then the usual questions come up: "Oh, does it hurt?" for example…and the trained employee can answer that perfectly, she or he now knows exactly what to say. And she is trained unconsciously in selling whitening.

So, where do you think most of these rich ladies will make the whitening? And where do you think they will send their husbands? That's the idea.

And on top of that, you can tell the owner, that you have an idea so that all the other employees are not angry. All the other employees of that place will get the bleaching for 50% off. And here again, we tell them that the owner is paying 50% of the whitening, and they have to pay the other 50%. And of course, you will train them the same way you trained the top employee.

IDEA #8: WEDDINGS (THE NOT-LOW-COST IDEA)

Weddings are a huge thing. Not only in Spain, but also in a lot of countries. At weddings they spend a lot of money in Spain, the average couple, not a rich couple, an average couple spends 25000 euros, in all together. In the restaurant, in the flowers, in the church, the invitation cards, the DJ the music, photography, the car, they hire to get them from the church to the restaurant, the honeymoon vacation all these things together. 25000 euros, the average. And worldwide, more than 50% of engaged women, who are not yet married, would whiten their teeth before the big day.

Where do they spend their money? They should spend it in your office. How do you get to these people?

You can cooperate with wedding agencies.
You can have a booth at a wedding fair.

<u>Cooperate with wedding agencies.</u>

You look for wedding agencies in your area. And then you talk to them, too. Because they organize the whole wedding for the usually rich people in your city. They do everything for them, starting from the dress, the flowers, and the menu, everything is organized.

You follow the same idea as in the strategic giveaway. You offer them a free whitening and then you talk to them. "Please incorporate some of my whitening, veneers, Invisalign™, and lip fillers, in the packages that you offer". Some of them have a premium package, a medium package, and a normal Package. The Premium Package is very comprehensive, so they usually are interested in getting related offers into that package. Whitening might be interesting for them to get it into the package, for a good deal.

You can talk to them about these options, and they will refer people to you that are going to marry. And by the way, the people that are going to marry, they fix their teeth and their mother wants to fix their teeth, too… and the mother-in-law also, believe me.

<u>Booth at a wedding fair</u>

This is the no-low-cost-idea. But it has brought my office a lot of patients, so the ROI (return on investment) was very good.

At the booth you can do several things:
Posters
Wedding-planner
Dice-game

There is very likely a wedding fair in your city or your area, and you can hire or rent a small booth. In the small booth, you will not only stay there and wait for people to come. They usually won't. That's what we did the first time. We waited, and people were walking around and never came to us. So we had to find out a way how to grab people's attention, with posters for example.

Show a **poster** with a bride and a gorgeous smile and put the text: "Go ahead! Have a really white wedding" referring to the teeth of the bride.

Another poster could be: 2x1, two for one, for whitening, only one of them, husband and wife, pays and both get the whitening for example.

This could be for couples, the parents, the best man, the friends, the guests, you can offer that to everybody. A wedding reaches a lot of people.

But they (both of them in the 2x1 offer) have to come in at once you have to explain the bleaching one time only. And they get the bleaching trays at the same time, you control them at the same time. You don't lose additional time with that.

Another idea for the wedding fair is a **wedding planner**. You can download that from the internet.

The wedding planners show the steps you have to take for a successful wedding. Like when it is the best time to look for a restaurant, when is the best time to look for a DJ, when is the best time to look for a hairdresser, photographer, and so on. It starts usually one year before the wedding. You can download that from the internet and then you put in different things when you, for example, should start a transparent aligner treatment to fix your teeth.

Six months before the wedding is a health-check of the teeth. Three months before the wedding, start a smile makeover for example, with veneers or something like that. One month before the wedding would be the last possible moment for that. Put this information inside this special wedding planner.

The last possible moment for a smile makeover with veneers is three weeks before the wedding. The last moment for take-home whitening is two weeks before a wedding. Last moment for an in-office whitening...., all these things can be put in between the steps the couple has to do before the wedding.

You print them with an online print service in a folded DIN A4 format, and then you give them away for free at your booth, you just have to remind yourself to put also your contact information on these small brochures.

And what has worked really well for us is this: We went and bought some dice. Big **dice**, like for babies to play with them.

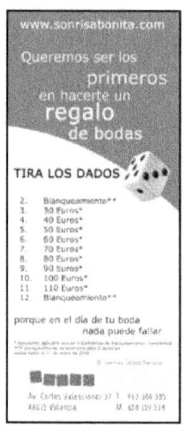

We bought two of them. You make a game with prices, the participants just throw them and if the combination is two (one and one) then they win a free whitening. If the combination is 12 (six and six) they win a free whitening, too. And all in between is a discount they get to spend on whitening. Imagine the combination is three and five, that's eight, then they have an 80 Euros discount on whitening. And they fill out cards with their name, email, and mobile phone number.

You can make this game and people come and play and then you say "Why don't you make it also for your future husband? Maybe he wins a free wedding and maybe he gives it to you? Who knows?" Then she throws the dice again, and she writes down the name and contact information of the future husband. You can go on with this strategy…."What about your mother? You don't think your mother can?"

And on your part, you write down who has won how much and they take the card with them. They can make an appointment right away at the booth with you. If they don't call you in the next week. You contact them and remind them of their prize.

You also go to other booths and offer to play the dice-game to the employees of the booths, the hostesses, they can also win a free whitening.

You can take a lot of advantage of going to a wedding fair, okay, but make it in a professional way and make it with some ideas of things that you give away. A wheel like this works, too.

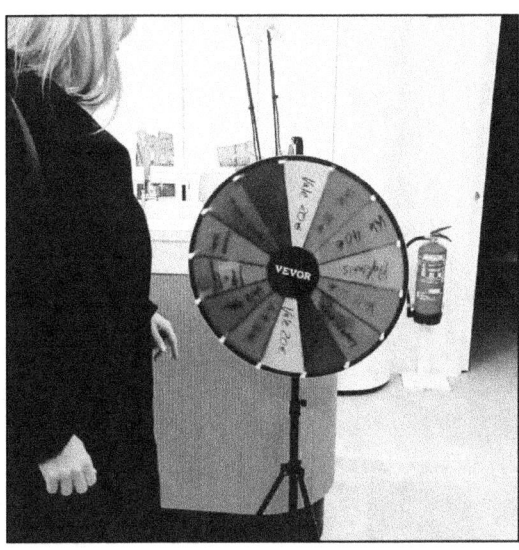

12
IDEA #9: SEND THEM THEIR BEFORE/AFTER

Sent the befores and afters to the patient. Always. And you better send them to their business email address or on a WhatsApp™.

If they are at their job place, and they receive that. Maybe they laugh a little bit or smile if they look at the pictures, and then their co-workers ask what happened.

And then your patient can say, "look, that's how I looked before". And then she or he shows how he looks now, and wow!

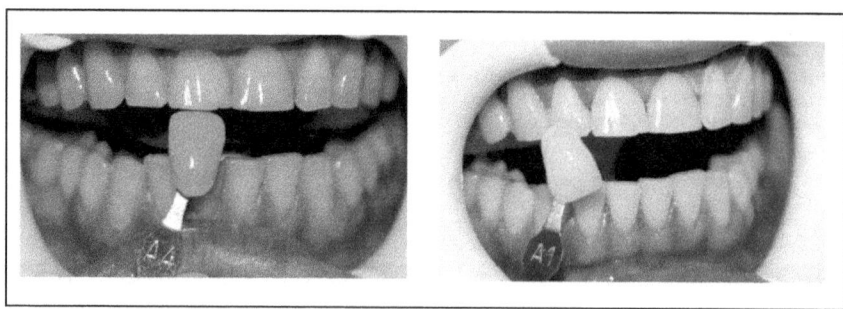

This starts a whole conversation on what has been done, and about you and your office. Form that habit, to take always before and after pictures of your patients, even with a simple whitening like this one.

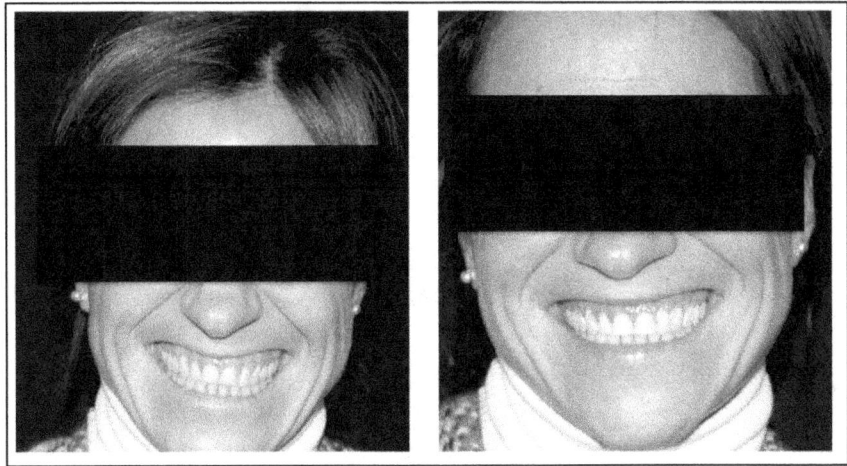

13
IDEA #10: OFFER SPECIAL HOURS

To have an advantage compared to your competitors, you need to offer something different than others. So, open in special hours.

For example, once a month, open on a weekend, or once a week, open two hours earlier than you would open normally. So, very early in the morning, once a week. These days you could close two hours earlier, too.

The same thing applies to very late in the evening and up to two hours later than you open normally.

This makes you different and this makes people, that are very comfortable with these office hours, come to you. They might not have time coming to your office because they are usually very busy. And if they are busy, they usually are busy making money.

They might have money to spend in your office, but they are not comfortable to come to your office during normal office hours. Sometimes people who make a lot of money are very busy. And they appreciate a lot these special hours.

You could even charge more for procedures done at these hours if you wish. You can charge a supplement during these hours if you want.

Nevertheless, it is very important that you have special hours available and you promote them over the internet the whole time. Use your channels to do so. Instagram, Facebook, Twitter, Homepage…..

14
IDEA #11: USE YOUR ELEVATOR PITCH

This chapter will talk about how to write your personal elevator pitch. And we will learn what it is and what it's not. You will learn the steps to write an elevator pitch, I will show you a template and an example of how to write your elevator pitch, and I will point out the mistakes you have to avoid.

You meet someone at the restaurant, in a networking event, in the gym, and they ask: What do you do for a living? Whatever you do, don't just say "I'm a dentist".

The response you'll usually get ranges from "Oh, I hate dentists" to "Does this look infected?". You don't want that.

Instead, see this as an opportunity to promote your skills and generate interest in the business world. This is called having an elevator pitch.

What is an elevator pitch? It is a powerful representation of who you are. It is a short, engaging introduction to you, and the value you offer.

And it tells someone why they should want to choose you as a dentist. What's the purpose? It is to quickly let others know what your expertise is, and what your greatest accomplishments are.

- It is very short.
- It is between 20 and 60 seconds. The best thing is under 30 seconds.
- It is goal-oriented.
- It is personal.
- It is about you. (It's not really about you, you will understand me later.) It's about what you can offer to others.
- It is specific and targeted.
- And It should be interesting.

What it should not be:
- It should not be a review of your resume.
- It should not be a list of your skills and strengths.
- And it should not be a request for a patient to come to your office.

He will naturally know that you are the correct person, and he will naturally choose you. It is more about what you have to offer to the listener.

It is not that you are a dentist. You should not say just that. But what should you say?

Lots of things get attention but only two things attract interest. You want to get the interest of the person that listens to you when you make that talk when you give that elevator pitch.

First of all, people are interested if they have a problem that they don't want, and a result they want, that they don't have. Let me repeat that.

People are interested when it comes to talking about a problem they have, they don't want, and about a result they want and they don't have.

If you have that in your elevator pitch, they are focused and they listen to you.

It is all about outcomes. Potential patients don't care about the work you do. They don't care about who you are. They don't care about how great you are. They only care about the outcome you can help them create. That's what they care about.

So, focus on the most awesome, most powerful outcome that you provide as a pure dentist, as an orthodontist, as an esthetic dentist, as a general dentist, as a pedodontist, or as a root canal specialist.

Build 100% of your messages, also the elevator pitch, around that. Advertisement, marketing, everything.

Step two, write your elevator pitch.

First, identify who you are, and whom you help.

Second, identify your why. Why you do what you do. Write that down. Write down whom you help, and write down why you do what you do. Your purpose, your passion, your commitment. Why you're passionate about what you do.

You will take elements of what you wrote down to make your elevator pitch. You can start with "One of my greatest passions is".

Third, what makes you unique or special? Your greatest accomplishments, the largest problems you have solved. Major contributions you have made, how many patients you have already treated? What's your background? Something special, something that makes you unique.

And fourth, after all, include a call to action. No elevator pitch without a call to action, or question at the end.

And then practice, practice, practice, practice, and revise and change. Don't be afraid to change it. Practice with family members, with friends, with colleagues.

Here is a template for your elevator pitch:

Hi, my name is X.

I'm an orthodontist, (dentist, periodontist, …) helping (the people you help and the pains you solve).

I'm passionate about X

I've been fortunate to (your biggest problems that you have solved or the greatest accomplishment that make you special)

Have you ever (then a question or a call to action)?

Let me show you an example.

"Hi, my name is Peter Smith.

I'm a smile-creating dentist helping people who are unhappy with the appearance of their teeth.

My greatest passion is to design and build the exclusive smiles of their dreams they love and enjoy.

I've been fortunate to have gone through years of aesthetic dentistry and dental implant training to be able to help over 5000 patients from all over the world to smile again.

Have you ever thought about enhancing your smile?"

This pitch is under 30 seconds and it is about really having all the elements of an elevator pitch you can change it towards your personal experience, and your personal situation.

And here is what you have to avoid:
- Speaking too fast. Yes, you only have 60 seconds or 30 seconds, but try to avoid cramming 15 minutes of information in about one minute.
- Using highly technical terms, acronyms, or slang. You want your pitch to be easily understood. Avoid using words that will confuse the average person. The last thing you want is that, whoever is listening to you, feels dumb.
- Not being focused. This isn't a general conversation, you're not discussing the weather. Keep your pitch clear and focused. Focus on what you do.
- Not practicing. First, write down your pitch. Read it over. Have your friends and family read it. Does it make sense?

Make sure it flows well and that there aren't any spots that feel rough or awkward. Then practice it, and practice it again. Keep practicing it until it becomes so easy for you to pitch that.

- Being too robotic. This is all about face-to-face interaction with someone you want to impress. Look for an easily approachable compensation style for your pitch.

- Not having a business card or other takeaway with you. Imagine you've sold them on yourself. They are convinced. Now how are they going to get a hold of you when they decide it's time to go into your office? Make sure you always have something on you to pass on that will allow people to not only remember you but contact you later.

Template for your Elevator Pitch

Hi, my name is Peter Smith

I am a smile creating dentist,

helping people who are unhappy with the appearance of their teeth

My greatest passion is to design and build the exclusive smiles of their dreams they love and enjoy

I´ve been fortunate to have gone through years of training in esthetic dentistry and dental implants to be able to help over 5000 patients from all over the world to smile again

have you ever thought about enhancing your smile?

15
IDEA #12: IMPROVE THE PATIENT EXPERIENCE

In this chapter, we will talk about how to improve the patient experiences in your office. Other than to reform and rebuilding your office (architecture), these tips are not expensive and can give you a competitive advantage.

In-Office Experiences

When a patient comes into your office, he starts to experience different things, our experiences are created and strengthened by diverse stimuli that help us absorb, interpret, and remember everything that we notice. Sights, scents, and sounds leave us with lasting impressions and long-term recognition.

We, as a dental office, have to play with that so that we can leave a footprint in the brain of the patient, a good footprint, that makes our office look very good inside of all the experiences that the patient has made.

We know, that we process visual material 60,000 times faster than text (Business2Community, 2014: http://www.business2community.com/marketing/power-visual-content-marketers-0924525).

And we know also, that music impacts the way we feel, act, and even think (Fast Company, 2013: http://www.fastcompany.com/3022942/work-smart/the-surprising-science-behind-what-music-does-to-our-brains).

We will have to play with visual material and sounds and music in our office.

We can create positive in-office experiences,
through architecture,
through scents,
through music,
through digital signature, and
through new technology.

Architecture

Get a facelift for your office. Make it look very appealing, make it look modern, light, and bright. Everything has to be clean and neat.

Consider a kid's corner and relaxing areas. Plan for a photo shooting corner also in the reception area, an area that is for selfies for the patients.

The reception area should be designed like an airline lounge with coffee and so on.

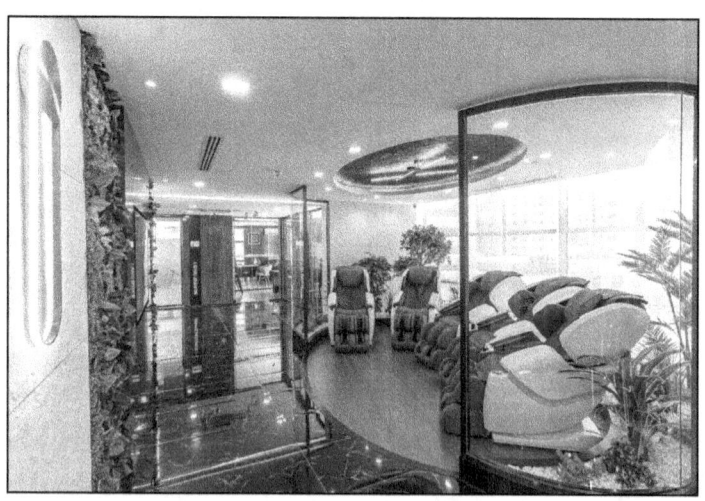

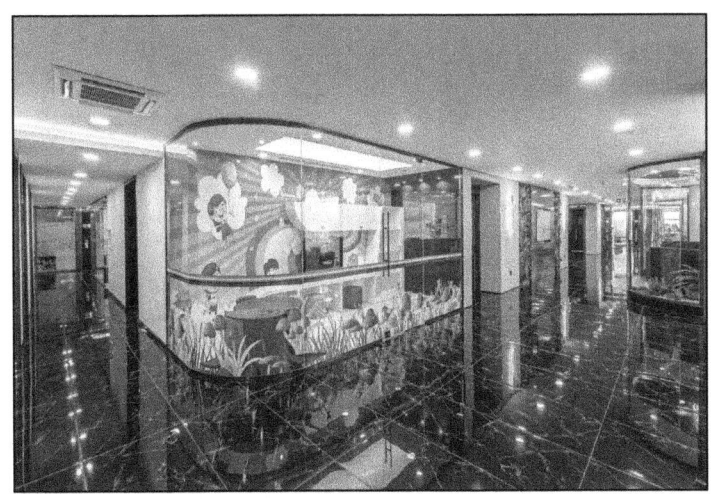

Here is, as an example, the DentSpa clinic in Istanbul Turkey. You see the relaxing areas and the kid's corner.

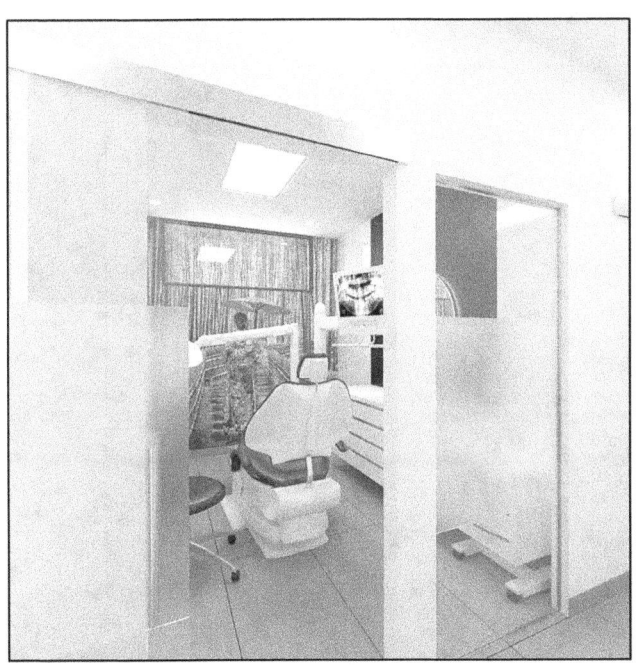

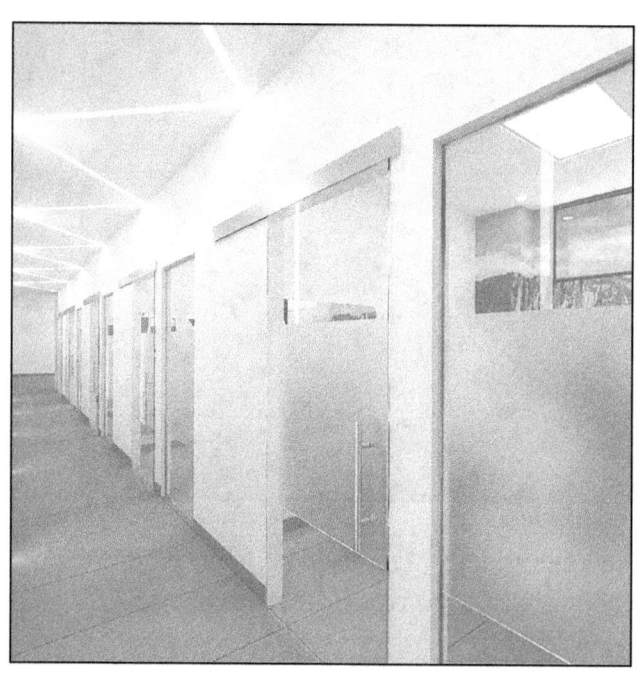

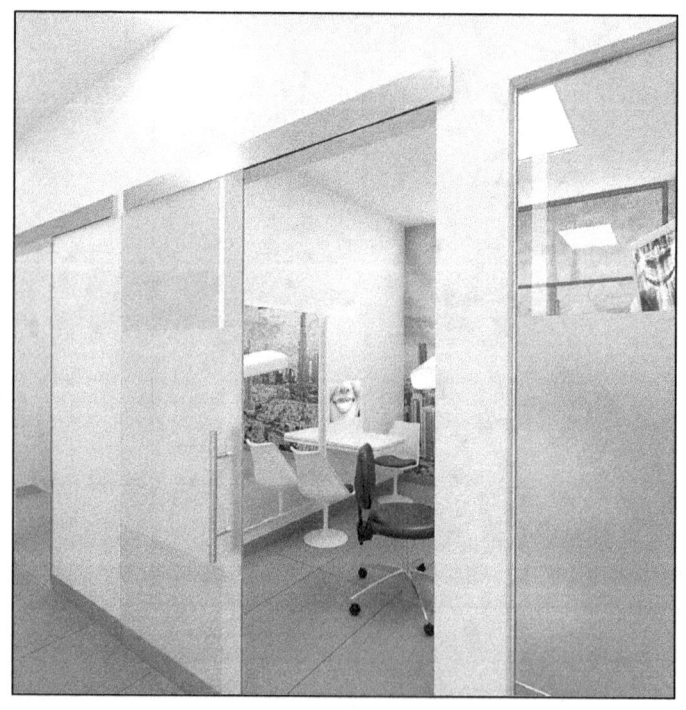

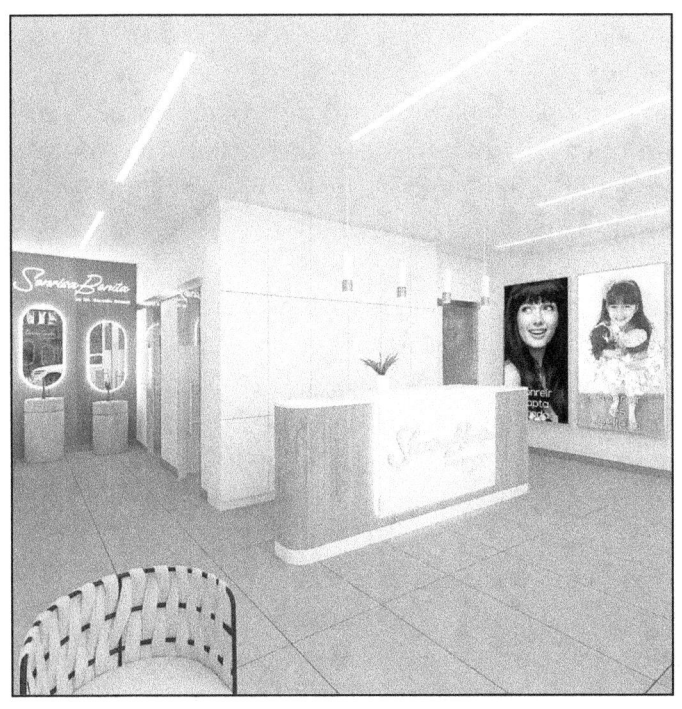

Here is an example from SonrisaBonita, in Valencia, Spain, my office. You see the outlet of the boxes, of the consultation rooms and you see that the patient is transferred to another area in this case to Kyoto, Japan. You see the area of the aisle, and you see the room Dubai, with a consultation corner. And you see the reception area with a corner to brush your teeth if you wish, before entering the treatment rooms.

Scents

The sense of smell is connected to the memory center, the limbic system of the brain. We connect positive and pleasant scents to positive memories. We want for sure, our patients to have positive memories of us.

People also connect unpleasant scents to negative memories, we do not want the patient to have unpleasant memories of us. Negative scents in a dental office would be formo-cresol, cresatin or metacresol, acrylic monomer, and eugenol. Also cleaning products, including antibacterial soap, disinfecting wipes, and even latex gloves.

Unpleasant odors come also from dental procedures, like fillings and root canals. In particular, the odor of the tooth dust created during the drilling of the teeth. We as dentists do not notice that, but the patient feels that a lot.

Since dental fears and phobias include fear of the smell of a dental office, combating unpleasant smells in dentistry should be a primary concern.

Fragrances have a beneficial effect on irritation, stress, depression, and apathy and enhance the positive factors of happiness, sensuality, relaxation, and stimulation.

The scent of a place is an effective differentiator.

You can create calming environments with scents, relaxing scents reduce patients' stress and you can create positive emotions. You get reduced cancellations if your office smells really good and you have also auto control. That means you control the bad odors, that come from your office. Scenting helps to eliminate or neutralize unpleasant odors and can also have anti-bacterial properties.

Relaxing scents more or less play around with lavender.

Vanilla has been used to decrease claustrophobia and tension.

Eucalyptus oils or rosemary and lavender can be used to treat malodors and have antibacterial properties.

Citrus scents are uplifting.

A good smell can improve a bad mood driving patients to be nicer to employees and vice versa.

Of course, the scents also affect our team.

Patients who are happy with the smell around them will likely be more open to considering additional services.

You might have different scents in your office for the reception area, the treatment rooms, and the toilets. People who walk into the front door, for example, are greeted with the warm cordial scent of sugar cookies. As people walk down the hall to the treatment rooms, the scent forms the experience from warm to relaxing with vanilla plus lavender scent for example.

The better your office smells, the more likely patients are to return and the scents are easy to install either in the ventilation system or in each room separately.

Music

Your In-Office experience can be enhanced through music. The music style and volume are very important. It introduces the vibe of the brand, of your brand. Your brand is the dental office. And the music style and volume also control the atmosphere and directly impact the psychology and habits of the patients.

63% of consumers have been influenced by a store's atmosphere. (The Marketing Site, 2015 http://www.themarketingsite.com/knowledge/7186/music-memory-and-retail-marketing).

Studies have found correlations between the type of music playing in the store and purchasing habits. In a wine retailer playing classical music instead of the top 40, for example, increased sales and led consumers to purchase more expensive bottles of wine. (Business Insider, 2011 http://www.businessinsider.com/effects-of-music-on-sales-2011-7?op=1).

In some countries, you can be liable for licensing violations if you play music from online channels like YouTube or other online channels. What you have to do is, to see what is the legislation in your country and then work accordingly to it.

When you play regular radio stations. Your music is constantly interrupted by advertisements, for example, maybe even advertisements from competitors playing in your office.

There are in store-music providers who can provide fully licensed music and selected playlists, that are carefully selected to enhance special feelings of well-being.

Digital signage

The next step is to enhance your in-office experiences through digital signage. If in-store music sets the tone of a store's atmosphere, then digital signals enhance it.

Digital signs are screens, that display custom text, videos, animations, and graphics. They are dynamic ways to convey information and engage patients in the clinic.

You can create content, that educates and informs, engages, entertains, promotes, and sells.

In the reception area, you can have big screens. In the treatment rooms also, but smaller screens. And at the reception desk, at the checkout, you can also have small screens like an iPad or something like that, a tablet where you can constantly display information and videos or pictures. In the toilets, you can also have some tablets. They're hung up and constantly giving information and entertaining the patient.

Also outdoors or on windows for people who walk by. These people then get that displayed information.

You can have signages in all these spaces, reception area treatment rooms, on the reception desk at checkout, toilets, and outdoors or windows. What kinds of devices? TV screens, tablets, LED panels, or even projectors.

The best digital signage content serves your business as well as your patients. Use your content to direct your patients to take action that will benefit them and your office. For example payment options, that the patient has, or new treatments that you are offering. Or let them know they should follow you on social media. Or inform them about complementary treatments like bleaching, fillers, lip fillers, or something like that.

Inform them about you, your team, treatments, new technology, special offerings or special opening hours, or special opening days they might not know about.

Financing options, promotions that you have, and before and after pictures.

You can also entertain with short funny scenes that you have done with your patients or with your team. Share patient testimonials and reviews.

Sometimes these videos are just displayed without sound. So you have to put the text that the patient says in a readable way. You can show ads for non-competing businesses for example.

Feature products or treatments, explain their value, and create urgency.

Introduce your staff, and promote events like an open day. Display date, time, and weather. Answer frequent ask questions through the screens.

New technology

You can enhance your in-office experience also through new technology, by displaying the new technology and showing the patient, that you have that new technology. Wi-Fi access, intraoral scanners, 3D printers, milling machines, and lasers.

If you have all this technology, the patient becomes aware of the fact, that he is in an up-to-date clinic and that he will be treated with the most modern treatment procedures.

Also cancer detection devices, like Velscope™ or ViziLitePRO™ for example, or microscopes. Digital Smile design software.

Not so new, but experience enhancing is nitrous oxide.

Also an oven for characterization of your milled crowns, so the patient sees that you are up to date the whole time.

Or even caries detection handpieces like the one from Lares™, where you can detect decay while you are drilling and you will just really eliminate the decay, and stop when you detect, that there is no decay anymore.

The new technology could also be teledentistry, that you offer on special hours on special days.

TV on the ceilings, video goggles for the patients, tablets for informed consent, or a patient fills out his data on the tablet directly.

Artificial intelligence. Like the Pearl software. The Second Opinion is a real-time radiographic detection aid. So, this program detects already some pathologies, or suggests that certain areas could have pathologies, and then you decide whether or not that's not a pathology or it is. So it can help you to detect or see things faster, easier, and better. We often look directly at the problem that we have at that moment. But somewhere else in the X-ray, there could be another problem we and the patient are not aware of, and we just don't have a glance at it. So this software can help us for example, and the patient sees: Wow, this doctor has the newest technology to be right on the top.

16
IDEA #13: STIMULATE REFERRALS

Stimulating referrals is a powerful marketing tool, as you use your own patients as ambassadors of your brand and office.

We will talk about how to stimulate referrals, what usually happens, some strategies to increase referrals, and how to handle a "no" if somebody doesn't want to refer to you.

What usually happens is, this: When you ask dentists, where most of their business comes from, they usually answer, that it's from referrals.

But most dentists' strategy is this: First, they hope, but hope is not a strategy. They hope, that people will talk about them, and people will refer to them.

Second, they might ask: "if you know somebody who needs my dentistry, please let me know". This is what they usually say to the patients. In this case, there is an action, which is good. But if the patient says, "I don't know anybody right now". Then what happens next? Nothing happens, nothing fast and continuous happens.

What strategies should you have?

Strategy number one:
Avoid the word referral when you are asking for referrals. Instead of using the word "referrals" use the word "introduce".

"Could you think of some friends, colleagues, or family that you could introduce to me?".

Strategy number two:
Ask for permission before you even treat them. The first time the patient comes in, you set the expectations. Your expectation is, that this patient as a new patient will refer to you patients later on. You can say that from the beginning of the relationship. "Mr. patient, my purpose is to help you to become so happy with the treatment, that you gladly would introduce me to at least three people you really care about" or "Mr. patient, I want you to be so delighted with the treatment, that at the end, I will ask you to introduce me to at least three people you really care about, does that seem fair enough?".

And then he knows, that you will do anything possible to make him happy, which is good. And in return, he gives you referrals. Of course, you would have tried to make him happy anyhow, but now he feels like he needs to give you something in return.

Now you have set the tone.

Strategy number three:
Imagine you have asked for advice instead of referrals. Imagine you have a highly successful patient. And you want more of these celebrities, soccer players, football players or basketball players or something like that.

Sometimes they're not comfortable being mentioned. They don't want you to mention them, because they have contracts with advertisement agencies. It happens to me a lot, by the way.

So, what do you do? If you ask directly, they feel uncomfortable, they don't like that usually. You have to apply another strategy.

You ask for advice in three steps.

Step number one: acknowledgment. What does that mean? "Mr. patient, I want to sincerely thank you for your confidence in us to help you design your new smile. And I'm truly grateful.".

You acknowledge a patient for being your patient and for his confidence.

Step number two: put him or her in your place. "Imagine you were me and run a dental office and you want to help more people like you, highly successful patients. And you would love to work with people who are introduced by good patients."

Step number three: ask for advice. "I'm curious what would a successful person like you do, to encourage people like you to introduce your friends, colleagues, and families to a dentist like me?".

These are highly successful people. They will come up with ideas on the spot so you just have to implement these ideas. And then you do it on them. So now it is difficult for them not to introduce you to their environment because it was *their* idea to proceed the way you are proceeding with them at that moment.

They gave you a tip on how to proceed, and you do it on them. Does it work? They told you, that this would work, so then they would have to refer patients to you.

Strategy number four:

What if the patient says "no, I don't want to refer"? Find out what has happened, and what has to happen. "Mr. patient, I would love to be the person whom you would feel comfortable introducing to your friends and family". Notice, we do not use the word refer. We use "introduce".

"Let me ask you a question. What should happen now, to make that a reality?" Take notes and let them talk. What has to happen?

Then "Mr. patient, let's pretend I do ABC, that you suggest. Would you be more comfortable to introducing two or three of your friends to us?" "Sure". That's it, you got it.

That's how you get referrals.
You don't hope you don't wait.

You proactively use words you use a script, the scripts in the strategies, that I just presented to you.

17
IDEA #14: GET CONVINCING PATIENT TESTIMONIALS

Patient testimonials are another powerful marketing tool at virtually zero cost. And you can use that piece of information in several formats.

Do you want to learn how to get perfect patient testimonials for your website and social media? Here, you will learn why testimonials are important and how to use them. And then the setup, how to do it, and the script of the best questions to get the most out of it. And then we will talk about the release and consent forms.

Why testimonials and how to use them? Well, people look you up online, before they call you. So prospective patients have zero idea what kind of clinician you are. They look for signs of familiarity and trust. Where do they find them? On the internet.

They insanely guess your clinical skills, by "feeling" whether or not your online reviews are legit. So they make conclusions, that are not at all logical.

It's all about the feeling they have about how good you are. So the most convincing piece of marketing they will see is a short clip of your current patients. And it's simply not good enough to say you are the best dentist in town, or that your crowns are the best. You need to prove it. And the best way to do this is for the satisfied patients to prove it for you.

Which patients should I ask for a testimonial? What kind of questions should I ask? How long should the videos be? What are the legal issues of the patient testimonials?

The patient is not sure where to start, and how to approach it. When you ask a patient to give you a testimonial, they don't know where to start and what to say. So, usually, you don't get very good testimonials. And either your practice gets sugary testimonials or no testimonials at all.

This is why you need to give them some guidelines. The guidelines are a list of questions that you have. And with this list, the patient can just answer these questions. Instead of coming up with something to tell about your office or you.

Your potential patients want to see someone who is just like them, recommending dental results, they hope to get themselves.
For this, the video is by far the best thing. You can use a video as a video, or you can use a video as audio. Or you can use the video as a written testimonial with or without a picture. You can use the whole clip or just a part of it as marketing material.

Keep in mind that this questionnaire is not for new patients. Ideally, this is for a raving fan of your office who has been through a lot with you and your staff. So let the patient choose which and how many questions he wants to answer. This gives you all sorts of different testimonials.

The best patients

The best patients for testimonials are

the ones who compliment you, or
the one who is a long-year patient, or
the one who has undergone a long treatment, or
the one who has achieved a good result, or
the one who refers a lot to you.

These are the best patients to ask for a testimonial.

The Setup

The Setup is easy and doesn't have to be expensive. You take your smartphone and put it horizontally, never vertically, always horizontally. And then you can buy a tripod, plus an LED ring-light for about 25 bucks at for example Amazon™.

And in any corner of your office or anywhere in your office, you can shoot.

Then you need editing software like iMovie™ or DaVinci Resolve™, which are also free. And if you do it professionally, you leave a space free next to the patient when you shoot the video to put a text either on the left or on the right side. This helps, to put the text or to highlight the words, or to put a word, that the patient is just saying at that moment.

Script of 17 best questions to get the most out of it

1) **Why did you trust our dental office with your oral health?**
Over 70% of people say they value a stranger's opinion when making a purchasing decision. By asking a question about why they chose to trust you and your services, you set yourself apart from your competitors.

2) As an alternative question to this question, you could ask: **What made you choose our dental office over others in the area?**

It points out your competitive differences. Maybe you are more conveniently located, offer more procedures, have longer opening hours, or offer the latest dental technology. But prospective patients aren't aware of this unless someone tells them.

3) What didn't you like about your smile before you came to us?

This connects your current patients to your potential patients, as they may have the same dental issue.

4) Alternative question to this question would be: **What was your initial dental problem?**

Maybe they didn't want a smile makeover. They were happy with their smile. But they had a dental problem.

The same thing, it connects your current patients to your potential patients, as they may have the same dental issue.

5) What did this dental problem prevent you from doing?

This gives motivation. If a potential patient can identify with the motivation for solving a dental problem, they will feel more in tune with the testimonial and it will be more powerful.

6) What made you decide to do something about your dental problem? And why now?

Same thing, it's a motivation for a potential patient to do something about it.

7) How did your recent dental procedure change that?

It shows that they have a problem and only you, as a dentist, can fix it.

8) What treatment did you have done?

It shows what treatment or treatments has or have been done on the patient.

9) **What was your favorite part about your patient experience in our dental office?**

You get a short clip, that can be used in any marketing. It doesn't matter if their favorite part was your friendly staff. Your quick treatment time, or the dentist's great chairside manner. It helps build social proof for your office.

10) An alternative question to this question would be: **What specifically do you like best about our dental practice?**

It gets patients thinking in terms of specific, and not bland generalities that could apply to any dental office. But it's specifically about your dental office. They start to think, about what specifically they like.

11) **How does the dental care you receive here differ from what you experienced in other dental offices?**

The patient might reveal stories about inadequate care as a child, unreasonable fears they had, or painful dental episodes. If they can explain how your office helped overcome these challenges, it might make it easier for the next patient, who may be experiencing similar concerns, to decide to come to you.

12) **What does our dental staff do, that makes you feel comfortable about coming here?**

It is aimed at all the prospects that have a fear of the dental office. If current patients can explain what makes them feel better, it might help someone else overcome their own fears. So, if they feel comfortable, maybe the new patient also will feel comfortable.

13) **How does your new smile make you feel?**

The most powerful piece of any marketing is the end result, or how it makes the patient feel. Your patients really don't go through teeth whitening to have whiter teeth. They whiten their teeth because they want to feel confident and beautiful.

How does everything make them feel? That is a purchasing motivation. It aims at their feelings.

14) **What is it that has kept you coming to our practice for so long?**
Testimonials from long-term patients are particularly valuable, as they point to a stable practice, that can build trust and confidence in the relationship. These patients feel strongly about the dental care they receive. You definitely want them to share that enthusiasm with others.

15) **What advice would you give other patients in a similar situation to you?** A simple command telling the possible new patient what to do. This ought to be a call to action along the lines of "I will just suggest anyone that feels like I did, contact the practice straightaway". So in the end this advice is a call to action to contact your office.

16) An alternative question to this question: **Would you recommend us to others you know? If so, why?**
Same thing. It is a call to action.

17) **Is there anything you would like to add?**
This gives them freedom in ideas and might reveal hidden things that you didn't think about, or that you did not consider important, but maybe mean a lot to that patient and perhaps also to possible future patients. Who knows?

You present a patient with this list of questions, and he can choose as many as he wants. And then you just ask these questions.
And the patient in front of the camera just answers the questions. That's it.

You need a release or consent form, and this release or consent form should contain certain things:

It should give you the right to use moving or still pictures and spoken words.

It should give you the right, that these statements may be used in printed publications, multimedia presentations, websites, or any other distribution media like social media, newspapers, radio, or television and

that the patient does not get any reimbursement for that testimonial.

You can download these release or consent forms for patient testimonials from the internet, but consider everything I just wrote about. It should be inside of that form, or just let a lawyer introduce these things to one you downloaded from the internet.

18
IDEA #15: OFFER MORE

Always give more.

Always offer more than people expect. Always deliver more than expected. Always deliver more than you promised.

If you promised 12 ideas, deliver 14 or 15. If you promise one thing, give more.

People who get what they expected, come back.

People who don't get what they expected, leave your office.

People who get more than they expected, become fans of your office and start to recommend you highly.

This is a good marketing tool for you. Go the extra mile. Incentive your employees to go that extra mile for the patients.

This is what you want to achieve.

19

OTHER BOOKS FROM THE AUTHOR

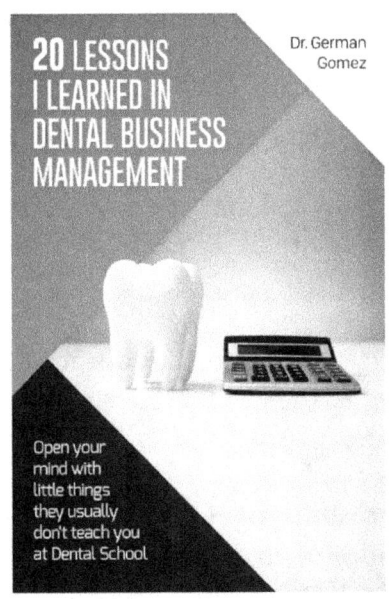

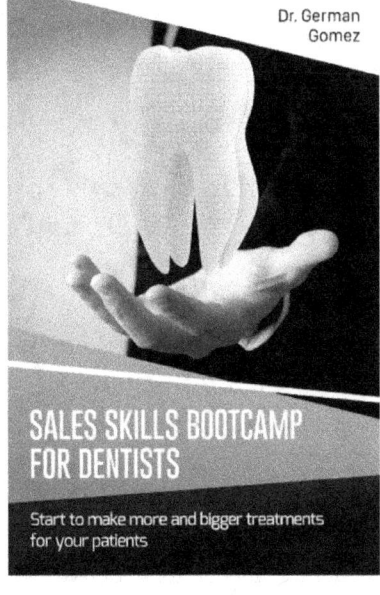

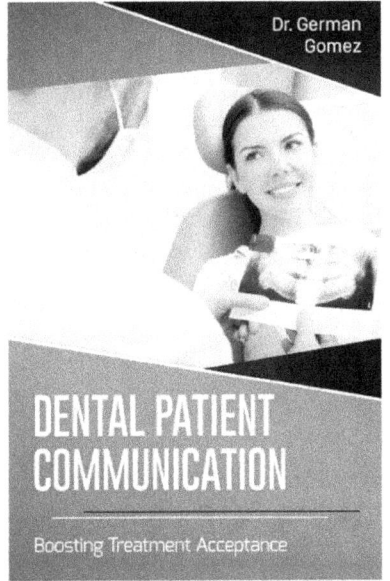

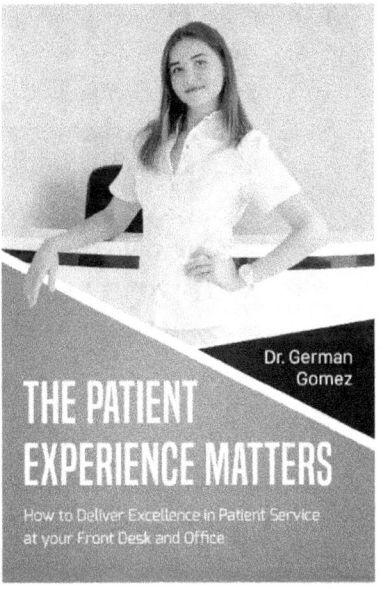

ABOUT THE AUTHOR

Dr. Gómez is Spaniard, born and grown up in Germany, and **D.D.S., M.D., and Ph.D.** from the University of Tübingen, **Germany**.

Since 1995, Dr. Gómez has been in **tight contact with the dental industry**. He worked in the headquarters of a big dental corporation for three years.

Since 1999, Dr. Gómez has held **over 480 lectures**, seminars, and hands-on workshops in 43 different countries all over the world, **many of them in Dental Business Management**.

After some years in the 5 most prestigious dental offices in Germany as an associate dentist, Dr. Gomez finally moved to Spain in 2004, where he runs his dental office in Valencia, Spain, focusing on **Esthetic Dentistry and Implants**. Over the years in Spain, he opened 3 different types of dental offices and closed two of them. A huge part of this experience is condensed in his books.

Spain is an extremely hostile environment to run a dental office as a business, due to the legislation and the overflow of dental universities. Starting from scratch and succeeding in that environment gives the book a higher value.